Healthy Instant Pot Cookbook

Easy Instant Pot Recipes for Keep Health and Lose Weight

Simon Tibbs

Sommario

Introduction

This complete and useful guide to instant pot cooking with over 1000 recipes for breakfast, dinner, supper, and even desserts! This is one of the most comprehensive instant pot cookbooks ever published thanks to its variety and accurate instructions.

Innovative recipes and classics, modern take on family's most loved meals – all this is tasty, simple and of course as healthy as it can be. Change the way you cook with these innovative instant pot instructions. Need a new dinner or a dessert? Here you are! Best instant pot meals come together in a few simple steps, even a beginner can do it! The instant pot defines the way you cook every day. This instant pot cookbook helps you make the absolute most out of your weekly menu.

The only instant pot book you will ever need with the ultimate collection of recipes will aid you towards a simpler and healthier kitchen experience. If you want to save time cooking meals more efficiently, if you want to offer your family food that can satisfy even the pickiest eater, you are in the right place! Master your instant pot and make your cooking needs fit into your busy lifestyle

Cayenne Eggs

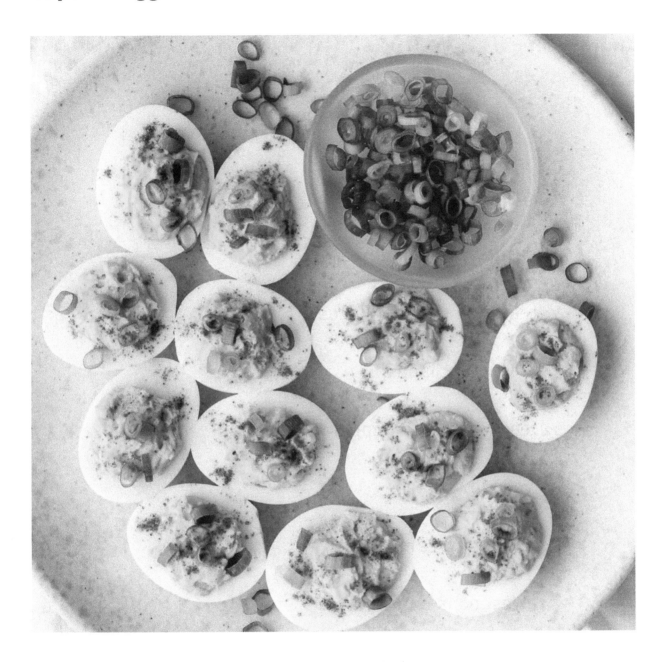

Prep time: 8 minutes

Cooking time: 7 minutes

Servings: 3

Ingredients:

- 4 eggs

- 1 teaspoon cayenne pepper

- ½ teaspoon red chili flakes

- ½ teaspoon cilantro

- ½ teaspoon white pepper

- 1 avocado, pitted

- ½ cup sour cream

- 2 tablespoons butter

- 3 tablespoons chives

Directions:

1. Combine the cayenne pepper, chili flakes, cilantro, and white pepper together. Mix up the mixture.

2. Chop the chives and slice the avocado.

3. Combine the sour cream and butter together. Blend the mixture until smooth.

4. Transfer the sour cream mixture in the pressure cooker. Add spice mixture.

5. Beat the eggs in the pressure cooker. Add chives and avocado and close the lid.

6. Set the pressure cooker mode to "Steam," and cook for 7 minutes. When the dish is cooked, remove it from the pressure cooker and serve it.

Nutrition: calories 410, fat 2, fiber 34.6, carbs 11.82, protein 15

Breakfast Strata

Prep time: 10 minutes

Cooking time: 15 minutes

Servings: 6

Ingredients:

- 6 slices keto bread

- 1 tablespoon mustard

- 1 teaspoon salt

- ½ cup parsley

- ¼ cup dill

- 1 cup cream

- 4 eggs

- 1 cup spinach

- 2 tablespoons butter

Directions:

1. Cut the keto bread into the cubes.

2. Transfer the half of the bread in the pressure cooker.

3. Whisk the eggs in the mixing bowl and add the salt, mustard, and cream.

4. Chop the spinach and parsley. Add the chopped greens in the egg mixture.

5. Add butter and whisk the mixture. Pour half of the egg mixture in the pressure cooker, and cover the dish with the remaining bread.

6. Add the second part of the egg mixture. Close the lid, and set the pressure cooker mode to "Steam." Cook for 15 minutes.

7. When the dish is cooked, allow it to cool briefly and transfer the dish to the serving plate. Cut it into pieces and serve.

Nutrition: calories 171, fat 10.3, fiber 3.2, carbs 11.9, protein 9.9

Cheddar Sandwiches

Prep time: 10 minutes

Cooking time: 10 minutes

Servings: 4

Ingredients:

- 8 slices keto bread

- 6 ounces ham

- 6 ounces cheddar cheese

- 1 tablespoon mustard

- 4 eggs

- 1 tablespoon mayonnaise

- 1 teaspoon basil

- 1 teaspoon cilantro

- ½ teaspoon ground black pepper

- 1 teaspoon paprika

Directions:

1. Slice the ham and cheddar cheese. Combine the mayonnaise, basil, cilantro, ground black pepper, and paprika together in a mixing bowl.

2. Add mustard and stir the mixture well. Spread every slice of bread with the mayonnaise mixture.

3. Add ham and cheddar cheese on the four of the bread pieces and cover that with the remaining bread pieces.

4. Whisk the eggs carefully, and dip the sandwiches in the egg mixture. Transfer the sandwiches to the pressure cooker and close the lid.

5. Set the pressure cooker mode to "Sauté," and cook for 10 minutes.

6. When the cooking time ends, remove the dish from the pressure cooker and serve immediately.

Nutrition: calories 399, fat 23.3, fiber 4.9, carbs 17.5, protein 31.3

Coconut Egg Toasts

Prep time: 10 minutes

Cooking time: 8 minutes

Servings: 7

Ingredients:

- 4 eggs

- 1 cup of coconut milk

- 3 tablespoons Erythritol

- 1 teaspoon vanilla extract

- 1 tablespoon butter

- 7 slices carb bread

Directions:

1. Beat the eggs in the mixing bowl and add coconut milk.

2. Whisk the mixture well and add Erythritol. Sprinkle the egg mixture with the vanilla extract and stir. Dip the bread slices into the egg mixture.

3. Add the butter in the pressure cooker.

4. Add the dipped bread slices and close the lid. Set the pressure cooker mode to "Sauté," and cook for 4 minutes on each side.

5. When the toasts are cooked, remove them from the pressure cooker and rest briefly before serving.

Nutrition: calories 175, fat 12.3, fiber 2.8, carbs 9.2, protein 8

Tortilla Breakfast Wraps

Prep time: 10 minutes

Cooking time: 10 minutes

Servings: 5

Ingredients:

- 5 almond flour tortillas

- 10 ounces ham

- 2 tomatoes

- 1 cucumber

- 1 red onion

- 1 tablespoon mayonnaise

- 2 tablespoons olive oil

- 2 tablespoons ketchup

- 1 teaspoon basil

- 1 teaspoon paprika

- ½ teaspoon cayenne pepper

- 4 ounces lettuce

Directions:

1. Slice the tomatoes and chop the cucumbers. Chop the ham.

2. Peel the red onion and chop it. Combine the mayonnaise, olive oil, ketchup, basil, paprika, and cayenne pepper and stir the mixture.

3. Spread the tortillas with the mayonnaise mixture and add chopped ham.

4. Sprinkle the dish with the chopped onion, sliced tomatoes, and chopped cucumbers. Add lettuce and wrap the tortillas.

5. Transfer the tortilla wraps in the pressure cooker and close the lid.

6. Set the pressure cooker mode at "Steam," and cook for 10 minutes.

7. Remove the dish from the pressure cooker and rest briefly.

Nutrition: calories 249, fat 15, fiber 4.1, carbs 14.7, protein 15.6

Banana Panini

Prep time: 5 minutes

Cooking time: 2 minutes

Servings: 4

Ingredients:

- 1 banana

- 8 slices low carb bread

- 2 tablespoons butter

- 1 teaspoon vanilla extract

- 1 teaspoon cinnamon

Directions:

1. Peel the banana and slice it. Spread bread with the butter from both sides.

2. Sprinkle the bread slices with the vanilla. Add banana and make sandwiches.

3. Transfer the sandwiches in the pressure cooker and close the lid.

4. Set the mode to "Sauté," and cook for 1 minute on each side.

5. Remove the sandwiches from the pressure cooker and rest briefly before serving.

Nutrition: calories 127, fat 6.4, fiber 3.1, carbs 14.3, protein 4.4

Chicken Balls

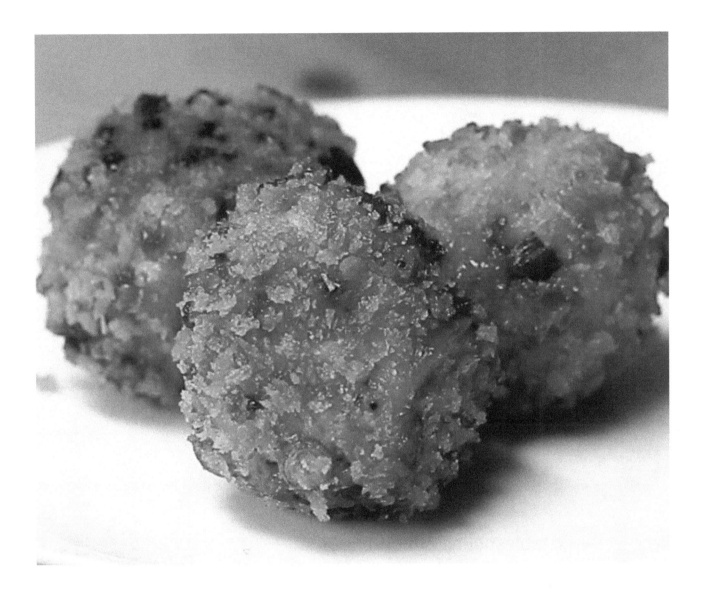

Prep time: 15 minutes

Cooking time: 30 minutes

Servings: 5

Ingredients:

- 5 eggs, boiled

- 1 cup ground chicken

- 1 teaspoon salt

- 1 teaspoon ground black pepper

- ½ cup pork rinds

- 1 teaspoon butter

- ½ teaspoon tomato paste

- 2 tablespoons almond flour

- 1 teaspoon oregano

Directions:

1. Peel the eggs. Combine the ground chicken, salt, ground black pepper, tomato paste, and oregano together in a mixing bowl.

2. Blend the mixture well. Make the balls from the ground chicken mixture and flatten them. Put the peeled eggs in the middle of the ball and roll the meat mixture around them.

3. Dip each one of them in the almond flour and pork rinds.

4. Add the butter in the pressure cooker and transfer the egg's balls. Close the lid, and set the pressure cooker mode to "Sauté."

5. Cook for 30 minutes.

6. Open the pressure cooker during the cooking to turn the balls.

7. When the egg balls are cooked, remove them from the pressure cooker and rest briefly. Serve immediately.

Nutrition: calories 237, fat 15.8, fiber 1.5, carbs 3.3, protein 21.6

Chorizo Topping

Prep time: 10 minutes

Cooking time: 8 minutes

Servings: 6

Ingredients:

- 8 ounces chorizo

- ⅓ cup tomato juice

- 1 teaspoon cilantro

- 1 tablespoon coconut flour

- 1 teaspoon olive oil

- 1 teaspoon butter

- 1 sweet bell peppers

- 3 eggs

- ⅓ cup of coconut milk

- 1 teaspoon coriander

- ¼ teaspoon thyme

- ⅓ cup fresh basil

Directions:

1. Combine the tomato juice, cilantro, coconut flour, olive oil, coriander, and thyme.

2. Stir the mixture well. Remove the seeds from the bell peppers and chop it.

3. Wash the fresh basil and chop it.

4. Add coconut milk in the tomato juice mixture and beat the eggs.

5. Blend the mixture using a hand mixer until smooth. Add the chopped peppers and butter. Chop the chorizo and add to the mixture.

6. Transfer the mixture to the pressure cooker and close the lid. Set the pressure cooker mode to "Steam," and cook for 6 minutes.

7. Open the lid and blend well carefully using a wooden spoon.

8. Close the pressure cooker lid, and cook for 2 minutes.

9. When the cooking time ends, let the dish rest briefly. Serve it immediately.

Nutrition: calories 260, fat 21.4, fiber 1.1, carbs 4.6, protein 12.7

Egg Muffins

Prep time: 10 minutes

Cooking time: 10 minutes

Servings: 6

Ingredients:

- 4 eggs

- ¼ cup almond flour

- 1 teaspoon salt

- ¼ cup cream

- 1 teaspoon baking soda

- 1 tablespoon lemon juice

- 1 white onion

- 5 ounces sliced bacon, cooked

Directions:

1. Beat the eggs using a whisk. Add almond flour and cream and whisk until smooth.

2. Peel the onion and dice it. Chop the cooked bacon.

3. Add the diced onion and chopped bacon in the egg mixture. Stir it carefully.

4. Add salt, lemon juice, and baking soda and stir the mixture.

5. Take muffin cups, and fill each one halfway with the egg dough.

6. Transfer the muffin cups in the pressure cooker basket and close the lid. Set the pressure cooker mode to "Pressure," and cook the muffins for 10 minutes.

7. When the muffins are cooked, remove them from the pressure cooker and rest briefly before serving.

Nutrition: calories 211, fat 15.7, fiber 0.9, carbs 3.6, protein 13.7

Cocoa Slow Cook

Prep time: 10 minutes

Cooking time: 13 minutes

Servings: 3

Ingredients:

- 1 cup flax meal

- 3 tablespoons cocoa powder

- 1 tablespoon Erythritol

- 1 teaspoon vanilla extract

- 1 cup of water

- ⅓ cup of coconut milk

- 1 tablespoon dark chocolate

- 1 tablespoon butter

- 1 teaspoon sesame seeds

- 3 tablespoons almonds

- 1 teaspoon raisins

- 1 teaspoon olive oil

Directions:

1. Crush the almonds. Combine the cocoa powder, Erythritol, vanilla extract, and chocolate together in a bowl and stir the mixture.

2. Spray the pressure cooker with olive oil.

3. Put the flax meal in the pressure cooker and add cocoa powder mixture. Add the crushed almonds, raisins, coconut milk, and water.

4. Blend the mixture using a wooden spoon. Close the pressure cooker lid, and set the mode to " Pressure." Cook for 13 minutes.

5. When the cooking time ends, mix up the carefully using a spoon until smooth. Transfer the cooked chocolate to serving bowls and serve.

Nutrition: calories 347, fat 30.3, fiber 13.9, carbs 19.7, protein 11.4

Breakfast Egg Muffins

Prep time: 10 minutes

Cooking time: 8 minutes

Servings: 5

Ingredients:

- 2 cup spinach, chopped

- 5 eggs, whisked

- 1 tablespoon flax meal

- ½ teaspoon salt

- 1 teaspoon turmeric

- ½ teaspoon butter

- 1 cup water, for cooking

Directions:

1. In the mixing bowl mix up together chopped spinach, whisked eggs, flax meal, salt, turmeric, and butter.

2. Transfer the mixture into the muffin molds. Pour water in the cooker and insert trivet. Place muffin molds on the trivet and close the lid.

3. Cook muffins for 8 minutes on High-pressure mode.

4. Then use quick pressure release. Chill the muffins until warm and remove from the muffin molds.

Nutrition: calories 77, fat 5.3, fiber 0.8, carbs 1.5, protein 6.2

Coconut Creamy Porridge

Prep time: 5 minutes

Cooking time: 10 minutes

Servings: 6

Ingredients:

- 1 cup chia seeds

- 1 cup sesame seeds

- 2 cups of coconut milk

- 1 teaspoon salt

- 3 tablespoons Erythritol

- ½ teaspoon vanilla extract

- 3 tablespoons butter

- 1 teaspoon clove

- ½ teaspoon turmeric

Directions:

1. Combine the coconut milk, salt, Erythritol, vanilla extract, clove, and turmeric together in the pressure cooker. Blend the mixture.

2. Close the lid, and set the pressure cooker mode to "Pressure."

3. Cook the liquid for 10 minutes. Open the lid and add chia seeds and sesame seeds.

4. Stir the mixture well and close the lid. Cook for 2 minutes.

5. Remove the dish from the pressure cooker and let it chill briefly before serving.

Nutrition: calories 467, fat 42.6, fiber 11.2, carbs 18.4, protein 9.3

Chicken Dill Quiche

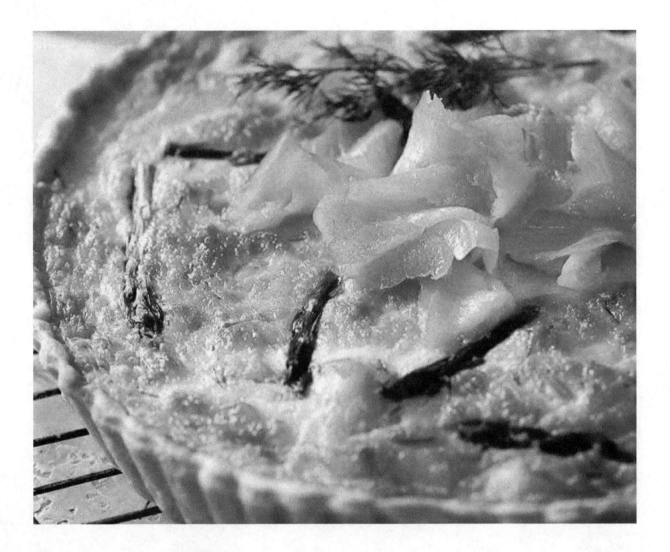

Prep time: 10 minutes

Cooking time: 30 minutes

Servings: 6

Ingredients:

- 1 pound chicken

- 1 cup dill

- 2 eggs

- 8 ounces dough

- 1 teaspoon salt

- ½ teaspoon nutmeg

- 9 ounces cheddar cheese

- ½ cup cream

- 1 teaspoon oregano

- 1 teaspoon olive oil

Directions:

1. Chop the chicken and season it with the salt, oregano, and nutmeg. Blend the mixture. Chop the dill and combine it with the chopped chicken.

2. Grate cheddar cheese. Take the round pie pan and spray it with the olive oil inside.

3. Transfer the yeast dough into the pan and flatten it well. Add the chicken mixture.

4. Whisk the eggs and add them to the quiche.

5. Sprinkle it with the grated cheese and add cream. Transfer the quiche to the pressure cooker and close the lid.

6. Set the pressure cooker mode to "Sauté," and cook for 30 minutes.

7. When the cooking time ends, remove the dish from the pressure cooker and chill it well. Cut the quiche into slices and serve it.

Nutrition: calories 320, fat 14.1, fiber 3, carbs 13.65, protein 34

Cardamom Chia Pudding

Prep time: 10 minutes

Cooking time: 15 minutes

Servings: 4

Ingredients:

- 1 cup chia seeds

- 4 tablespoons Erythritol

- 2 cups of coconut milk

- 2 tablespoons heavy cream

- 1 teaspoon butter

- 1 teaspoon cinnamon

- 1 teaspoon ground cardamom

Directions:

1. Combine the chia seeds, Erythritol, and coconut milk together in the pressure cooker.

2. Stir the mixture gently and close the lid. Set the pressure cooker mode to "Saute" and cook for 10 minutes.

3. When the cooking time ends, let the chia seeds rest little.

4. Open the pressure cooker lid and add cream, cinnamon, cardamom, and butter. Blend the mixture well using a wooden spoon.

5. Transfer the pudding to the serving bowls. Add cherry jam, if desired, and serve.

Nutrition: calories 486, fat 43.3, fiber 15.3, carbs 22.6, protein 8.8

Creamy Soufflé

Prep time: 10 minutes

Cooking time: 20 minutes

Servings: 6

Ingredients:

- 3 eggs

- 1 cup cream

- 6 ounces of cottage cheese

- 4 tablespoons butter

- ⅓ cup dried apricots

- 1 tablespoon sour cream

- 2 tablespoons sugar

- 1 teaspoon vanilla extract

Directions:

1. Whisk the eggs and combine them with cream.

2. Transfer the cottage cheese to a mixing bowl, and mix it well using a hand mixer.

3. Add the whisked eggs, butter, sour cream, sugar, and vanilla extract.

4. Blend the mixture well until smooth.

5. Add the apricots, and stir the mixture well.

6. Transfer the soufflé in the pressure cooker and close the lid. Set the pressure cooker mode to «Sauté», and cook for 20 minutes.

7. When the cooking time ends, let the soufflé cool little and serve.

Nutrition: calories 266, fat 21.1, fiber 1, carbs 11.72, protein 8

Zucchini Casserole

Prep time: 10 minutes

Cooking time: 30 minutes

Servings: 8

Ingredients:

- 6 ounces cheddar cheese

- 1 zucchini

- ½ cup ground chicken

- 4 ounces Parmesan cheese

- 3 tablespoons butter

- 1 teaspoon paprika

- 1 teaspoon salt

- 1 teaspoon basil

- 1 teaspoon cilantro

- ½ cup fresh dill

- ⅓ cup tomato juice

- ½ cup cream

- 2 red sweet bell peppers

Directions:

1. Grate cheddar cheese.

2. Chop the zucchini and combine it with the ground chicken.

3. Sprinkle the mixture with the paprika, salt, basil, cilantro, tomato juice, and cream. Stir the mixture well. Transfer it to the pressure cooker.

4. Chop the dill, sprinkle the mixture in the pressure cooker, and add the butter. Chop the Parmesan cheese and add it to the pressure cooker.

5. Chop the bell peppers and add them too. Sprinkle the mixture with the grated cheddar cheese and close the lid.

6. Set the pressure cooker mode to "Sauté", and cook for 30 minutes.

7. When the cooking time ends, let the casserole chill briefly and serve.

Nutrition: calories 199, fat 14.7, fiber 1, carbs 6.55, protein 11

Spinach Casserole

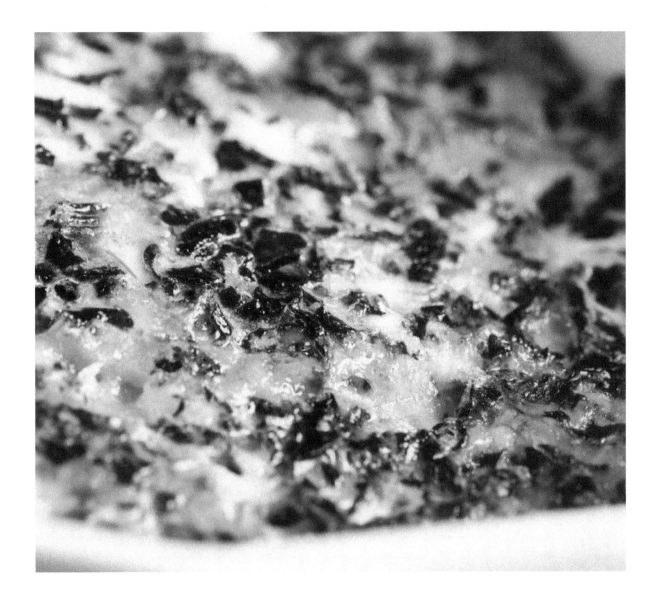

Prep time: 6 minutes

Cooking time: 6 minutes

Servings: 5

Ingredients:

- 2 cups spinach

- 8 eggs

- ½ cup almond milk

- 1 teaspoon salt

- 1 tablespoon olive oil

- 1 teaspoon ground black pepper

- 4 ounces Parmesan cheese

Directions:

1. Add the eggs to a mixing bowl and whisk them.

2. Chop the spinach and add it to the egg mixture.

3. Add the almond milk, salt, olive oil, and ground black pepper. Stir the mixture well. Transfer the egg mixture to the pressure cooker and close the lid.

4. Set the pressure cooker mode to "Steam," and cook for 6 minutes.

5. Grate the cheese. When the cooking time ends, remove the omelet from the pressure cooker and transfer it to a serving plate.

6. Sprinkle the dish with the grated cheese and serve.

Nutrition: calories 257, fat 20.4, fiber 0.9, carbs 3.4, protein 17.1

Spicy Romano Bites

Prep time: 6 minutes

Cooking time: 20 minutes

Servings: 8

Ingredients:

- 10 ounces Romano cheese

- 6 ounces sliced bacon

- 1 teaspoon oregano

- 5 ounces puff pastry

- 1 teaspoon butter

- 2 egg yolks

- 1 teaspoon sesame seeds

Directions:

1. Chop Romano cheese into small cubes.

2. Roll the puff pastry using a rolling pin. Whisk the egg yolks.

3. Sprinkle them with the oregano and sesame seeds.

4. Cut the puff pastry into the squares, and place an equal amount of butter on every square. Wrap the cheese cubes in the sliced bacon.

5. Place the wrapped cheese cubes onto the puff pastry squares. Make the "bites" of the dough and brush them with the egg yolk mixture.

6. Transfer the bites in the pressure cooker.

7. Close the lid, and set the pressure cooker mode to "Steam." Cook for 20 minutes.

8. When the cooking time ends, remove the dish from the pressure cooker and place on a serving dish.

Nutrition: calories 321, fat 24.4, fiber 1, carbs 10.9, protein 16

Eggs and Chives

Prep time: 4 minutes

Cooking time: 4 minutes

Servings: 3

Ingredients:

- 3 eggs

- 6 ounces ham

- 1 teaspoon salt

- ½ teaspoon ground white pepper

- 1 teaspoon paprika

- ¼ teaspoon ground ginger

- 2 tablespoons chives

Directions:

1. Take three small ramekins and coat them with vegetable oil spray.

2. Beat the eggs add an equal amount to the ramekins. Sprinkle the eggs with the salt, ground black pepper, and paprika.

3. Transfer the ramekins to the pressure cooker and set the mode to "Steam."

4. Close the lid, and cook for 4 minutes. Meanwhile, chop the ham and chives and combine them.

5. Add ground ginger and stir into the ham mixture well. Transfer the mixture to the serving plates.

6. When the cooking time ends, remove the eggs from the pressure cooker and put them atop the ham mixture.

Nutrition: calories 205, fat 11.1, fiber 1, carbs 6.47, protein 19

Zucchini Quiche

Prep time: 15 minutes

Cooking time: 40 minutes

Servings: 6

Ingredients:

- 3 green zucchini

- 7 ounces puff pastry

- 2 onions

- 1 cup dill

- 2 eggs

- 3 tablespoons butter

- ½ cup cream

- 6 ounces cheddar cheese

- 1 teaspoon salt

- 1 teaspoon paprika

Directions:

1. Wash the zucchini and grate the vegetables.

2. Peel the onions and chop them. Grate the cheddar cheese.

3. Whisk the eggs in the mixing bowl. Roll out the puff pastry.

4. Spread the pressure cooker basket with the butter and transfer the dough to there.

5. Add grated zucchini and chopped onions, and sprinkle the vegetable mixture with the salt and paprika.

6. Chop the dill and add it to the quiche. Sprinkle the dish with the grated cheese and egg mixture, and pour the cream on top.

7. Close the pressure cooker lid, and set the mode to "Steam."

8. Cook the quiche for 40 minutes.

9. When the cooking time ends, check if the dish is cooked and remove it from the pressure cooker. Let the dish cool briefly and serve.

Nutrition: calories 398, fat 28.4, fiber 2, carbs 25.82, protein 12

Almond Pumpkin Cook

Prep time: 10 minutes

Cooking time: 15 minutes

Servings: 5

Ingredients:

- 1 cup almond milk

- 1 cup of water

- 1 pound pumpkin

- 1 teaspoon cinnamon

- ½ teaspoon cardamom

- ½ teaspoon turmeric

- ⅓ cup coconut flakes

- 2 teaspoons Erythritol

Directions:

1. Peel the pumpkin and chop it roughly.

2. Transfer the chopped pumpkin in the pressure cooker and add almond milk and water. Sprinkle the mixture with the cinnamon, cardamom, turmeric, and Erythritol.

3. Add coconut flakes and stir the mixture well.

4. Close the pressure cooker lid, and set the mode to "Sauté." Cook for 15 minutes.

5. When the cooking time ends, blend the mixture until smooth using a hand blender.

6. Ladle the pumpkin in the serving bowls and serve.

Nutrition: calories 163, fat 13.5, fiber 4.5, carbs 13.1, protein 2.3

Tomato Omelet

Prep time: 8 minutes

Cooking time: 9 minutes

Servings: 6

Ingredients:

- 5 eggs

- ½ cup of coconut milk

- 4 tablespoons tomato paste

- 1 teaspoon salt

- 1 tablespoon turmeric

- ½ cup cilantro

- 1 tablespoon butter

- 4 ounces Parmesan cheese

Directions:

1. Whisk the eggs with the coconut milk and tomato paste in the mixing bowl.

2. Add salt and turmeric and stir the mixture. Grate the Parmesan cheese and add it to the egg mixture.

3. Mince the cilantro and add it to the egg mixture. Add the butter in the pressure cooker and pour in the egg mixture.

4. Close the pressure cooker lid, and set the mode to "Steam."

5. Cook for 9 minutes. Open the pressure cooker to let the omelet rest. Transfer it to serving plates and enjoy.

Nutrition: calories 189, fat 14.6, fiber 1.2, carbs 4.9, protein 11.7

Poached Eggs with Paprika

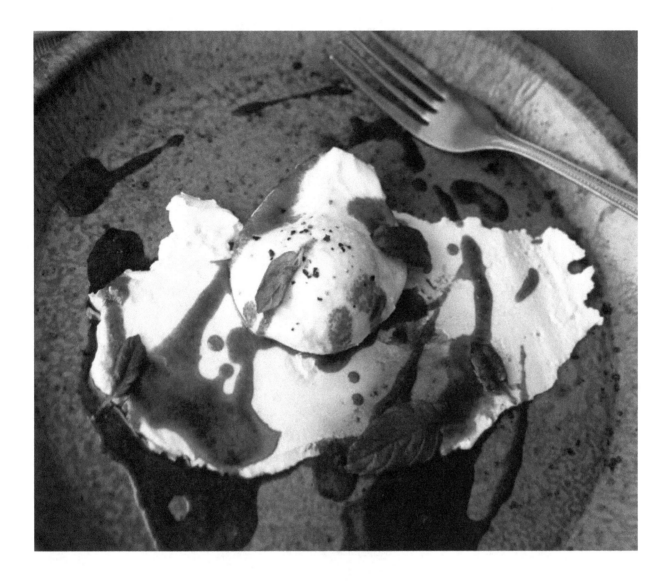

Prep time: 5 minutes

Cooking time: 5 minutes

Servings: 4

Ingredients:

- 4 eggs

- 3 medium tomatoes

- 1 red onion

- 1 teaspoon salt

- 1 tablespoon olive oil

- ½ teaspoon white pepper

- ½ teaspoon paprika

- 1 tablespoon fresh dill

Directions:

1. Spray the ramekins with the olive oil inside. Beat the eggs in a mixing bowl and add an equal amount to each ramekin.

2. Combine the paprika, white pepper, fresh dill, and salt together in a mixing bowl and stir the mixture.

3. Dice the red onion and tomatoes and combine. Add the seasonings and stir the mixture.

4. Sprinkle the eggs with the tomato mixture. Transfer the eggs to the pressure cooker.

5. Close the lid, and set the pressure cooker mode to "Steam". Cook for 5 minutes.

6. Remove the dish from the pressure cooker and rest briefly. Let it rest for a few minutes and dish immediately.

Nutrition: calories 194, fat 13.5, fiber 2, carbs 8.45, protein 10

Flax Mix

Prep time: 10 minutes

Cooking time: 25 minutes

Servings: 6

Ingredients:

- ½ cup flax seeds

- ½ cup flax meal

- ½ cup sunflower seeds

- 1 tablespoon tahini paste

- 3 cups chicken stock

- 1 teaspoon salt

- 1 onion, diced

- 3 tablespoons butter

- 3 ounces dates

Directions:

1. Combine flax seeds, flax meal, and sunflower seeds together in a mixing bowl. Add salt and diced onion.

2. Chop the dates and add them to the mixture. Transfer the mixture in the pressure cooker and add chicken stock.

3. Blend the mixture and close the lid. Set the pressure cooker mode to "Saute" and cook for 25 minutes.

4. When the cooking time ends, remove the mixture from the pressure cooker, and transfer it to a mixing bowl. Add butter and stir. Transfer the dish to serving plates.

Nutrition: calories 230, fat 15.7, fiber 7.3, carbs 19.4, protein 5.9

Scotch Turmeric Eggs

Prep time: 15 minutes

Cooking time: 30 minutes

Servings: 4

Ingredients:

- 4 eggs, boiled

- 1 cup ground beef

- 1 teaspoon salt

- 1 teaspoon turmeric

- 1 teaspoon cilantro

- ½ teaspoon ground black pepper

- ½ teaspoon butter

- 1 tablespoon lemon juice

- ½ teaspoon lime zest

- 1 tablespoon almond flour

- ⅓ cup pork rinds

- ¼ cup cream

Directions:

1. Peel the eggs. Combine the ground beef, salt, turmeric, cilantro, ground black pepper, lemon juice, and lime zest together. Stir the mixture well.

2. Make the medium balls from the meat mixture and flatten them well. But the peeled eggs in the middle of the flatten balls and roll them.

3. Dip the balls in the almond flour. Dip the meatballs in the cream and sprinkle them with the pork rind. Transfer the balls to the pressure cooker and close the lid.

4. Set the pressure cooker mode to "Sauté," and cook for 30 minutes.

5. When the cooking time ends, remove the scotch eggs from the pressure cooker carefully and serve immediately.

Nutrition: calories 230, fat 13, fiber 0.4, carbs 1.8, protein 25.8

Salty Broccoli Rice

Prep time: 10 minutes

Cooking time: 15 minutes

Servings: 4

Ingredients:

- 2 cup of broccoli rice

- 4 cups of water

- 1 tablespoon salt

- 3 tablespoons heavy cream

Directions:

1. Combine the broccoli rice, salt, and water together in the pressure cooker. Add cream.

2. Stir the mixture gently and close the lid. Cook for 15 minutes on the mode to "Saute"

3. When the broccoli rice is cooked, remove it from the pressure cooker and rest briefly.

4. Transfer the dish to the serving bowl. Serve the dish only warm.

Nutrition: calories 54, fat 4.3, fiber 1.2, carbs 3.3, protein 1.5

Breakfast Pasta Casserole

Prep time: 10 minutes

Cooking time: 20 minutes

Servings: 6

Ingredients:

- 6 ounces Palmini pasta, cooked

- 8 ounces Romano cheese

- 1 cup cream

- 3 tablespoons butter

- 1 teaspoon salt

- 1 teaspoon paprika

- 1 teaspoon turmeric

- 1 cup parsley

- 1 teaspoon cilantro

Directions:

1. Grate the cheese. Place pasta in the pressure cooker.

2. Sprinkle it with half of the cheese. Chop the parsley and add it in the pressure cooker mixture.

3. Season the mixture with the salt, paprika, turmeric, and cilantro. Sprinkle the casserole with the remaining cheese.

4. Add the butter and cream and close the lid. Set the pressure cooker mode to "Pressure," and cook for 20 minutes.

5. When the casserole is cooked, remove it from the pressure cooker and cut into serving pieces.

Nutrition: calories 256, fat 18.5, fiber 1.9, carbs 6.7, protein 17.5

Pumpkin and Raisins Puree

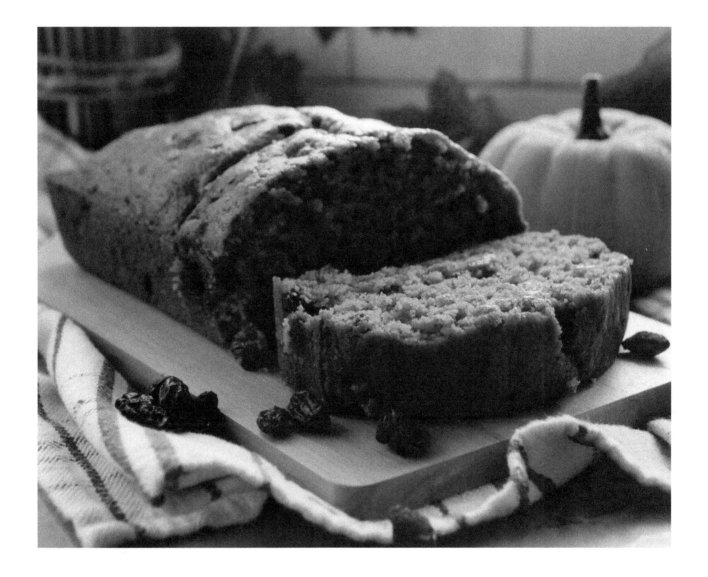

Prep time: 10 minutes

Cooking time: 20 minutes

Servings: 5

Ingredients:

- ¼ cup raisins

- pound pumpkin

- ½ cup of water

- 1 teaspoon butter

- tablespoons heavy cream

- 1 teaspoon cinnamon

- ½ teaspoon vanilla extract

- 1 tablespoon liquid stevia

Directions:

1. Peel the pumpkin and chop it. Transfer the chopped pumpkin in the pressure cooker. Add water, butter, cinnamon, and vanilla extract.

2. Close the lid and cook for 20 minutes at the pressure cooker mode to "Pressure".

3. When the cooking time ends, remove the mixture from the pressure cooker, and transfer it to a blender.

4. Blend it well until smooth.

5. Add raisins and cream and stir mixture well. Add liquid stevia and stir it again.

6. Chill the puree briefly and serve.

Nutrition: calories 82, fat 3.3, fiber 3.1, carbs 13.7, protein 1.4

Cauliflower and Tomato Balls

Prep time: 10 minutes

Cooking time: 20 minutes

Servings: 4

Ingredients:

- 1 pound cauliflower

- 1 white onion

- 3 tablespoons coconut flour

- 1 teaspoon olive oil

- ¼ cup tomato juice

- 1 teaspoon salt

- 2 tablespoons flax meal

- 1 teaspoon chicken stock

- 2 eggs

Directions:

1. Chop the cauliflower roughly and transfer it to a blender.

2. Peel the onion and chop it. Transfer the chopped onion in a blender. Add the flax meal and eggs to a blender and blend on high until smooth.

3. Remove the mixture from a blender and add chicken stock, salt, and flour. Knead the smooth cauliflower dough.

4. Make the small balls from the cauliflower mixture and transfer them to the pressure cooker. Add tomato juice and close the lid.

5. Set the pressure cooker mode to "Steam," and cook for 20 minutes.

6. When the cooking time ends, unplug the pressure cooker and leave the cauliflower balls to rest for 10 minutes.

7. Remove the dish from the pressure cooker and transfer it to serving plates.

Nutrition: calories 121, fat 5.3, fiber 6.7, carbs 14.1, protein 6.9

Almond Yogurt

Prep time: 10 minutes

Cooking time: 30 minutes

Servings: 6

Ingredients:

- 8 cups almond milk

- 2 tablespoons plain Greek yogurt

Directions:

1. Pour the almond milk in the pressure cooker and close the lid.

2. Set the pressure cooker mode to "Steam" and cook the milk for 30 minutes or until it is reached 380 degrees Fahrenheit.

3. Remove the milk from the pressure cooker and chill it until it reaches 100 F.

4. Add the plain Greek yogurt and blend well.

5. Let the mixture chill in the refrigerator overnight.

6. Stir the yogurt carefully using a wooden spoon and transfer it to serving bowls.

Nutrition: calories 82, fat 3.4, fiber 0, carbs 10.8, protein 1.4

Vanilla Bread Pudding

Prep time: 10 minutes

Cooking time: 30 minutes

Servings: 7

Ingredients:

- 1 cup cream

- ½ cup of coconut milk

- 10 slices low carb bread

- 2 tablespoons butter

- 1 teaspoon vanilla extract

- 3 eggs

- 1 teaspoon salt

- 4 tablespoons stevia powder

Directions:

1. Chop the bread in the medium cubes and transfer it to the pressure cooker.

2. Combine the coconut milk and cream together. Add eggs and whisk the mixture using a hand mixer.

3. Add the vanilla extract, salt, and stevia. Stir the mixture well.

4. Pour the mixture in the pressure cooker and close the lid. Leave the mixture for 15 minutes to let the bread absorb the coconut milk liquid.

5. Set the pressure cooker mode to "Pressure," and cook for 30 minutes.

6. When the cooking time ends, open the pressure cooker lid and let the pudding rest.

7. Transfer the dish to serving plates.

Nutrition: calories 255, fat 15.4, fiber 6.1, carbs 13.7, protein 17.4

Cauliflower Mac Cups

Prep time: 10 minutes

Cooking time: 25 minutes

Servings: 6

Ingredients:

- 8 ounces cauliflower, chopped

- 1 cup cream

- 1 cup of water

- 3 tablespoons butter

- 1 teaspoon salt

- 1 teaspoon basil

- 6 ounces Romano cheese

- 1 teaspoon paprika

- 1 teaspoon turmeric

- 3 ounces ham

Directions:

1. Coat six ramekins with butter. Combine the cauliflower, cream, and water together in a mixing bowl. Add salt, basil, paprika, and turmeric.

2. Chop the ham and Romano cheese. Add the chopped ingredients in the cauliflower mixture and stir it well.

3. Separate the cauliflower mixture between all ramekins and transfer the ramekins to the pressure cooker.

4. Close the lid, and set the pressure cooker mode to "Steam." Cook for 25 minutes.

5. When the dish is cooked, it should have a creamy, soft mixture, then let it cool briefly and serve.

Nutrition: calories 221, fat 17, fiber 1.3, carbs 5.3, protein 12.6

Flax Meal with Flakes

Prep time: 10 minutes

Cooking time: 7 minutes

Servings: 3

Ingredients:

- 1 cup flax meal

- 3 cups of coconut milk

- 2 tablespoons Erythritol

- 1 teaspoon vanilla extract

- 3 tablespoons almond flakes

- ½ teaspoon cinnamon

- ½ teaspoon nutmeg

Directions:

1. Put the flax meal in the pressure cooker and add coconut milk.

2. Sprinkle the mixture with Erythritol, vanilla extract, cinnamon, and nutmeg.

3. Blend the mixture well until smooth.

4. Close the pressure cooker lid, and set the pressure cooker mode to "Steam". Cook for 7 minutes.

5. Open the pressure cooker lid and stir the carefully. Transfer it to serving bowls and sprinkle with the almond flakes.

Nutrition: calories 739, fat 72.4, fiber 16.6, carbs 25, protein 14.2

Zucchini Pasta with Chicken

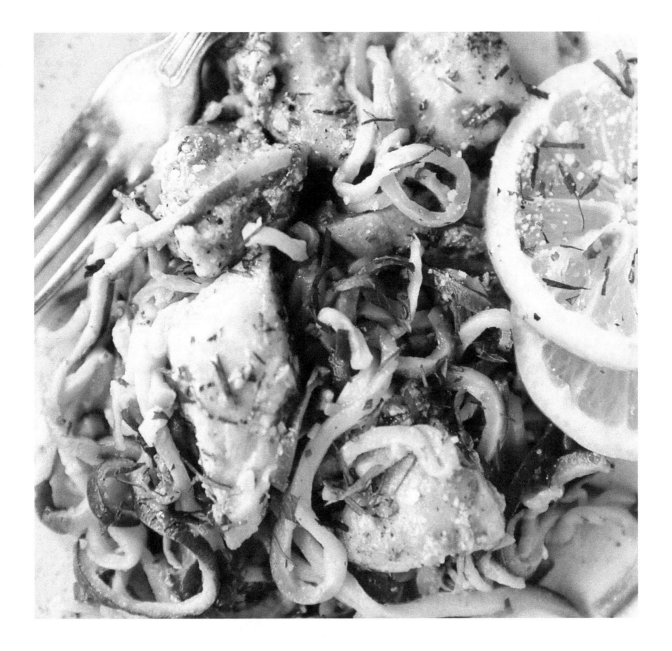

Prep time: 10 minutes

Cooking time: 25 minutes

Servings: 5

Ingredients:

- 1 zucchini

- 1 cup ground chicken

- ½ cup cream

- ½ cup chicken stock

- 1 teaspoon salt

- 1 teaspoon ground black pepper

- 1 teaspoon paprika

- ½ teaspoon ground coriander

- 1 teaspoon cilantro

- 1 onion

Directions:

1. Wash the zucchini and peel the onion. Grate the vegetables and combine them together in a mixing bowl.

2. Add ground chicken, cream chicken stock, salt, ground black pepper, paprika, ground coriander, and cilantro.

3. Blend the mixture well, and transfer it to the pressure cooker. Close the lid, and set the pressure cooker mode to "Sear/Sauté." Cook for 25 minutes.

4. Open the pressure cooker lid and stir. Transfer the dish to the serving bowl and chill well.

Nutrition: calories 87, fat 3.6, fiber 1.2, carbs 4.7, protein 9.2

Grated Zucchini Scramble

Prep time: 10 minutes

Cooking time: 6 minutes

Servings: 2

Ingredients:

- ½ zucchini, grated

- 2 eggs, whisked

- 1 teaspoon butter

- ¼ cup cream

- 1 teaspoon ground black pepper

Directions:

1. Preheat cooker on Saute mode and toss butter. Melt it and add grated zucchini.

2. Sprinkle the vegetables with ground black pepper and cream. Stir well.

3. Cook them for 3 minutes.

4. Then add whisked eggs and cook for 1 minute.

5. Scramble eggs and cook them for 2 minutes more.

6. Close the cooker and switch off it. Let the scramble rest for 10 minutes.

Nutrition: calories 110, fat 8.1, fiber 0.8, carbs 3.6, protein 6.5

Eggs Soufflé

Prep time: 10 minutes

Cooking time: 45 minutes

Servings: 4

Ingredients:

- 8 ounces of cottage cheese

- 4 eggs

- ½ cup cream

- 4 tablespoons butter

- 3 tablespoons Erythritol

- 1 teaspoon vanilla extract

Directions:

1. Pour the cream into the pressure cooker basket and close the lid.

2. Set the pressure cooker mode to "Stew" and cook the dish until the cream rich the temperature of 180 F (approximately 20 minutes).

3. Meanwhile, combine the cottage cheese and eggs together. Add Erythritol, vanilla extract, and butter. Blend the mixture using a hand blender.

4. Add the cottage cheese mixture in the preheated cream mixture.

5. Stir it carefully until smooth.

6. Close the lid and cook the dish on the yogurt mode for 25 minutes.

7. Remove the dish from the pressure cooker and rest briefly. Serve the soufflé warm.

Nutrition: calories 362, fat 28.3, fiber 0, carbs 12.99, protein 14

Coconut Porridge with Milk

Prep time: 10 minutes

Cooking time: 20 minutes

Servings: 5

Ingredients:

- 1 cup chia seeds

- ⅓ cup raisins

- ½ cup coconut cream

- 2 tablespoons butter

- ½ teaspoon ground ginger

- 1 teaspoon vanilla extract

- 1 cup almond milk

- 2 tablespoons Erythritol

Directions:

1. Combine the coconut cream and almond milk together, and add ground ginger, vanilla extract, and Erythritol. Stir the mixture well.

2. Add the butter and stir the mixture again.

3. Chop the raisins.

4. Transfer the coconut cream mixture in the pressure cooker.

5. Add chia seeds and chopped fruit. Stir it.

6. Close the lid, and set the pressure cooker mode to "Slow cook" Cook for 15 minutes.

7. When the porridge is cooked, open the pressure cooker lid and stir the dish gently. Transfer the dish to the serving bowls.

Nutrition: calories 266, fat 19.1, fiber 10.7, carbs 21.2, protein 5.6

Cheddary Beef Sandwich

Prep time: 10 minutes

Cooking time: 12 minutes

Servings: 2

Ingredients:

- 1 cup minced beef

- ½ teaspoon chili flakes

- 1 tablespoon water

- ½ teaspoon garlic powder

- ¼ teaspoon salt

- 2 eggs, beaten

- 2 cheddar cheese slices

- 1 teaspoon butter

Directions:

1. In the mixing bowl combine together the minced beef, chili flakes, water, salt, and garlic powder.

2. Then make 4 meatballs and press them gently with the help of the fingertips.

3. Wrap every ball in paper foil.

4. Pour water in the instant pot and insert the steamer rack.

5. Place the meatballs on the rack and cook them on Manual (high pressure) for 8 minutes.

6. After this, remove the meatballs from the instant pot and remove them from the paper foil.

7. Clean the instant pot and remove the steamer rack.

8. Preheat the instant pot on Saute mode and add butter.

9. Melt it.

10. Add beaten egg and cook them for 2 minutes. Then flip on another side.

11.   Place the one slice of cheese in the center egg and wrap it.

12.   Repeat the same steps with remaining cheese and egg.

13.   Then place the first wrapped cheese on 1 meatball and cove rit with the second meatball to get the sandwich.

14.   Repeat the same steps with the remaining ingredients.

15.   Pierce the cooked sandwiches with toothpicks if needed.

Nutrition value/serving: calories 353, fat 20.9, fiber 0.1, carbs 1.2, protein 38.5

Keto Walnuts Bowl

Prep time: 10 minutes

Cooking time: 10 minutes

Servings: 2

Ingredients:

- 1 tablespoon flaxseeds

- 1 tablespoon sesame seeds

- ¼ cup walnuts, chopped

- ¼ cup almonds, chopped

- ¼ teaspoon ground cinnamon

- ½ teaspoon vanilla extract

- 1 tablespoon coconut oil

- 1 egg white, whisked

Directions:

1. In the mixing bowl combine together flaxseeds, sesame seeds, walnuts, almonds, ground cinnamon, and vanilla extract.

2. Then add coconut oil and whisked egg white.

3. Mix up the mixture.

4. Preheat the instant pot on Saute mode.

5. Then place the nut mixture in the instant pot bowl and flatten it gently.

6. Cook the cereals for 10 minutes. Stir them every 2 minutes.

7. Then cool the cereals well.

Nutrition value/serving: calories 281, fat 25.3, fiber 4.2, carbs 6.6, protein 9.5

Butter Crepes

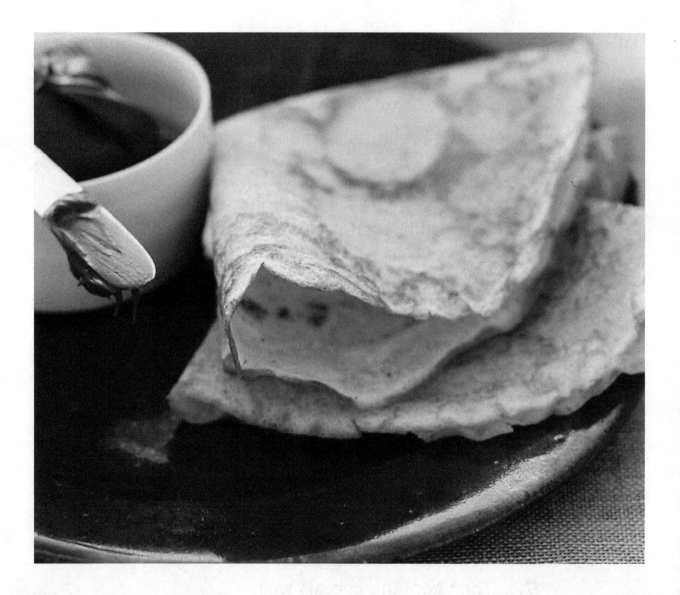

Prep time: 10 minutes

Cooking time: 15 minutes

Servings: 4

Ingredients:

- ½ cup of coconut milk

- 1 egg, beaten

- 1 tablespoon butter, melted

- ½ teaspoon baking powder

- 1 teaspoon lemon juice

- 1 teaspoon vanilla extract

- ½ cup almond meal

- 4 tablespoons ground coconut flour

- ½ teaspoon coconut oil, melted

- ¼ teaspoon salt

Directions:

1. In the mixing bowl mix up together coconut milk, eggs, melted butter, baking powder, lemon juice, vanilla extract, and salt.

2.   Then add the almond meal and ground coconut flour.

3.   Stir the mixture until you get the thick liquid.

4.   Grease the instant pot bowl with coconut oil.

5.   Preheat the instant pot on Saute mode for 3 minutes.

6.   After this, ladle 1 ladle of the crepe batter in the instant pot bowl in the shape of crepe.

7.   Cook the crepe on Saute mode for 1 minute from each side. Cook the crepes additional time if you prefer the golden-brown crust.

8.   Repeat the same steps with the remaining crepe batter.

Nutrition value/serving: calories 204, fat 17.8, fiber 2.8, carbs 8.4, protein 5.2

Pepper Eggs

Prep time: 10 minutes

Cooking time: 4 minutes

Servings: 2

Ingredients:

- ¼ teaspoon ground black pepper

- ¼ teaspoon salt

- ½ teaspoon butter, melted

- 2 eggs

- 1 cup water, for cooking

Directions:

1. Pour water in the instant pot and insert the steamer rack.

2. Place the eggs on the rack and close the instant pot lid.

3. Cook the eggs on Manual mode (Low pressure) for 4 minutes.

4. Then cool the eggs in the ice water and peel them.

5. Cut the eggs into halves and sprinkle with salt, ground black pepper, and melted butter.

Nutrition value/serving: calories 72, fat 5.3, fiber 0.1, carbs 0.5, protein 5.6

Conclusion

Being an excellent option both for immediate pot newbies and experienced instant pot users this instantaneous pot cookbook boosts your everyday cooking. It makes you appear like a professional as well as cook like a pro. Thanks to the Instantaneous Pot component, this cookbook aids you with preparing straightforward and also delicious meals for any kind of budget plan. Satisfy every person with hearty suppers, nutritive breakfasts, sweetest treats, as well as enjoyable treats.

Regardless of if you cook for one or prepare bigger sections-- there's a service for any kind of feasible cooking circumstance. Enhance your methods on exactly how to cook in the most reliable means utilizing only your immediate pot, this recipe book, and some perseverance to find out quick.

Valuable ideas and techniques are subtly integrated right into every dish to make your family members request new dishes over and over again. Vegetarian choices, options for meat-eaters and also very pleasing concepts to join the entire family members at the very same table. Consuming in your home is a common experience, as well as it can be so good to satisfy all together at the end of the day.

Master your Immediate Pot and make the most of this brand-new experience beginning today!

CPSIA information can be obtained
at www.ICGtesting.com
Printed in the USA
LVHW061218110521
687091LV00008B/1395